THE THREE DAY WAY

TO BETTER FITNESS

AND NUTRITION

FOR MEN & WOMEN

By Paul J. Godfrey

ISBN: 0-75964-064-5

This book is printed on acid free paper.

1stBooks – rev. 7/5/01

CONTENTS

PART I

PART II

ACKNOWLEDGEMENTS

To my family for being supportive.

To Professional wrestler Henry Roy for having confidence in me.

To my friends, who are ready and willing to try new ideas.

To Peter Mastrangelo and to Bruno Ragnacci for being supportive.

To Nyota Nayo for being confident and supportive.

To all of my clients who have experimented with this program and achieved great results.

To my lawyer Richard Cardali for being supportive.

To my lawyer friend Tina R. Newsome for being supportive.

PREFACE

As a Medical Doctor and Participant in weight training and nutrition, I am particularly impressed with Paul Godfrey's Weight Training and Nutrition Program.

With it, he has created a system that is safe, simple and effective.

The Program outlined in this book, when followed exactly, will give the individual an impressively tight, toned body without a bulky look.

By using the basic principles of bodybuilding and combining them with nutrition, Paul has created a system that will cause an increase in muscle tone and energy.

For years people have complained about not having time to workout due to late hours at the office, traveling, or working two jobs. This is why

Paul has come up with ideas about training routines that will save time.

INTRODUCTION

Most people are in pretty good shape, but the fact is many people are not dedicated to putting the time in for the results they want, when it comes to any sort of training programs.

Another element is the pain that comes along after the body has been worked out thoroughly, like the myth saying of "no pain no gain". This is true because muscle tissue heats up quickly and causes a burning sensation.

When it comes to small parts like calves, forearms and/or trapezius muscles they are normally more difficult to build unless you're gifted.

Without proper nutrition and guidance on fitness training, workout efforts will be limited because fat would cover the developing muscles.

Injuries will be enhanced more when training is done incorrectly.

Throughout these chapters you will learn the correct way to eat an stay fit with weight training and freehand exercises.

Both routines will give you a well toned look. No body parts should be overtrained, this will bring on excessive soreness to the muscle tissue and delay your progress. This is why the proper guidance is needed.

PART I

Paul J. Godfrey

CHAPTER ONE

WHAT ARE FREE WEIGHTS?

Free weights are barbells and dumbbells used to build and tone your muscles; (invented many years ago) and with continued research and study there is also the discovery of steel weights, sand, water, chrome and rubber weights.

Free weights will benefit you with great results regardless of what they are made of. The reason being, weight is weight and resistance is resistance. The big difference is when there's a push or pull movement. The same matter goes for training done with free weights.

****

HOW TO USE FREE WEIGHTS

Free weights should be used with caution:

If you have never done any physical activity before, check with your doctor for a physical prior to proceeding with your training.

Free weights should be used three (3) times a week for anyone just beginning a training program. For example: Monday - Wednesday - Friday or Tuesday - Thursday - Saturday.

In order to make your workout simple, you should familiarize yourself with the following terms:

EXERCISE TERMINOLOGY:

1. **Exercise**:A particular movement that is performed in order to develop a specific muscle. For example, the barbell curl is a biceps exercise.

2. **Set**: A number of repetitions performed without stopping.

3. **Rest:** A pause between sets; the rest enables you to gather strength for your next set.

4. **Routine:** All of the exercises performed for a particular body part on a given day. For example, Monday: - should routinely consist of two exercises: A standing barbell press and a seated barbell press.

5. **Workout:** The total of all exercises performed on a given day. For example: - Your workout will consist of your entire chest, shoulders and triceps routines. You will have performed two exercises for each of these body parts, and you will have performed three (3) sets of ten (10) repetitions each for every exercise.

CHAPTER TWO

MUSCLE DESCRIPTION

This chapter will help you understand the muscle groups and how they function.

1. **Chest:** The muscles located under your breasts which are fanlike in shape are called pectorals. They work to move your arms. They consist of two muscle groups, upper and medial.

2. **Shoulders:** These muscles are technically called deltoids. They are three headed muscles that are held to raise the arms. The three heads are front or anterior muscles which work as you move your arms in a forward direction; side or medial muscles, which help to move your arms out to the sides; rear or posterior muscles which

work to move your arms in a backwards direction.

3. **Triceps:** Triceps are a three-headed muscle that consists of an inner, outer and medial head. All three heads of the muscle are attached to the shoulder blade. Its job is to extend the forearm and arm, and to help pull back the arm once it is extended.

4. **Biceps:** The biceps is a two headed muscle that originates in the shoulder blade and ends in the forearm. The biceps work to bend or flex the arm at the elbow.

5. **Back:** The back muscles are the latissimus dorsi, or lats which provide the "V" shape to the back when properly developed. The other

back muscles are the trapezius and the upper back muscles. The two large trapezius muscles run on either side of the spine from the back of the neck to the middle of the back. They work to support the head and shoulders. The lats are used to help pull the shoulder back and the arm toward the body.

6. **Thighs**: The front thigh is called the quadriceps muscle because it consists of four muscles that travel along the front thigh and end in the kneecap. These muscles work to extend the leg from a bent position. The back thigh or biceps femoris hamstrings are made up of three muscles that are located on the back outside of the thigh and insert through the inside of the knee. These muscles work

together to rotate the leg, extend the hips, and flex the knee.

7. **Buttocks:** The buttock muscle is called the gluteus maximus because it is the largest muscle in the body. It runs from the hipbone to the tailbone, and works to extend and rotate the thigh.

8. **Abdominals:** The abdominal muscle is called the rectus abdominis. It is a single long, slender muscle that rises from the ribs near the breastbone and runs vertically along the abdominal wall. The abdominal area is divided into two parts, upper and lower. The abdominal muscles work to pull the torso toward the lower body.

9. **Calves**: The calf muscles are comprised of the gastrocnemius and the soleus muscles. The gastrocnemius is divided into two parts, which connect in the middle of the lower leg and tie in with the achilles tendon. The job of the gastrocnemius muscle is to flex the knee and foot downward. The soleus muscle is located underneath the gastrocnemius muscle. It assists the gastrocnemius in flexing the foot downward.

CHAPTER THREE

TO BUILD PREWORKOUT ENERGY

The idea is to have enough carbohydrates in your body; about an <u>hour</u> or <u>two</u> before training. (Example): Carb drink, Protein drink, or an energy bar low in fat. This way the body is not too sluggish which will cause slow digestion. The body should also have a good amount of water before, during and after training.

After training it is necessary to have a carb drink to replace the nutrients that were lost during training.

DESIGNING A BALANCED DIET

In designing a diet it is necessary to know the persons blood pressure, body weight, body fat, temperature, number of calories expended during exercise and the individuals life style and taste. This information is fed into a computer and it analyzes the values and tells you what the person needs to eat and what to avoid; also the menu proportions. For example, try this three square meal plan:

Breakfast

1 cup oatmeal

3 egg whites

1 bran muffin (or) 2 pieces whole wheat toast

orange juice (or) water/green tea

"No Time" — 1 cup plain yogurt, 8 oz. orange juice, & 1 banana — mixed in blender.

Lunch

Salad/soup

Turkey/tuna sandwich, lettuce, tomatoes (no mayo)

Water (or) green tea

Dinner

4 oz. fish/chicken breast

1 potato white (or) sweet with a 6 oz. green vegatable.

**NOTE: Dring 64 oz. of water daily.

CHAPTER FOUR

WHO CAN USE THESE WORKOUT TECHNIQUES?

1. Men and women with the desire to become tight and toned.

2. Anyone who wants increased strength and coordination.

3. Anyone who likes to workout at home or while traveling.

4. Anyone who has sustained an injury to a particular body part and wants to rehabilitate it.

5. Anyone who trains at a gym.

How long will it take to see results?

Within three (3) to six (6) months you'll actually begin to see result. Your body will feel tighter, stronger and more fit; you will also feel more equalized and stimulated.

DON'T THINK OF SKIPPING A WORKOUT

1. If you're thinking of skipping a workout it will delay your goals to achieve your level of excellence.

2. It will also change the appearance of your physical structure if you continue to skip workouts.

3. If you feel lazy, or pressed for time do some free hand exercises, as illustrated in the following chapters.

WHAT YOU CAN ACHIEVE WITH A PROGRAM OF REGULAR EXERCISE

If you exercise faithfully with the correct form, you should notice an increase in strength and coordination within a short time. Your flexibility will be better, you'll use less energy in performing both physical and mental tasks. You'll have better posture, you'll be able to reduce stress and tension, your heart should become stronger and your circulation improve. You'll have greater immunity from illness. You'll be better protected from injuries and be able to heal more rapidly when one does occur. You'll have greater immunity from illness. You'll be better protected from injuries and be able to heal more rapidly when one does occur.

GET A CHECKUP PRIOR TO BEGINNING A TRAINING PROGRAM

You may look great, feel great, but before anyone over the age of 25 engages in any form of strenuous exercise, including tennis, football, jogging, a medical checkup is advisable. The doctor will probably give you a go-ahead.

If you have some health problems, he can take proper measures to correct it. I think a physical exam is important; not only will you find out whether or not your heart is sound, but you'll also be checked for other conditions you might have such as: Vitamin deficiency, low metabolism rate, thyroid problems. These are things that affect how you lose or gain weight. They could put you off balance (equilibrium) and make you body fail to respond favorably although you are training hard, eating right and getting sufficient sleep.

If you are physically active and in reasonably good health, you can start your weight-training program.

ANALYZE YOURSELF

Before you start working out, it's important to look at yourself and categorize ourself in terms of which of the three body types you are. Most people are a combination of characteristics from more than one type, but the dominant characteristics are what you should be looking for in your assessment.

1. <u>The Ectomorph</u>:   A thin person with a light bone structure and long tenuous muscles. The ectomorph has a tough time gaining weight and building strength.

2. <u>The Endomorph</u>:   A stocky person with thick bones and a general tendency to be round and stout.   The endomorph will gain fast and be able to handle heavy training. His body is more likely to remain block and muscular without showing great cuts or definition.

3. <u>The Mesomorph</u>: Anatomically, the ideal body for weight resistance training. The mesomorph has a large frame and the capacity for becoming muscular fast.

You can improve your body. All that you should look for in training with weights is that you should 100% of your potential. That potential varies greatly among three body types and individuals within each type. If you are a skinny guy, an ectomorph, you are not really lost, though your kind of muscles are the most difficult to build, you may need to change your metabolism and perhaps correct a problem with your thyroid gland so you can start gaining weight - so, in a way, you're on the safe side.

If you're an endomorph, one of those round people who really have muscle tone to begin with, you should realize you won't have it as hard as the ectomorph, but you'll need to put more mental energy into it than the muscular type mesomorph.

CHAPTER FIVE
WHAT IS CARDIOVASCULAR?

Cardiovascular exercise is an essential part of any fitness program; it aids in weight loss, reduces the risk of heart disease and increased endurance and energy levels. Before doing any weight training it is essential to do some sort of warmup exercises to prevent injuries. The following are some good cardiovascular warm ups: Jogging in place, running on the treadmill and/or stationary biking.

Cardiovascular exercise is done by all athletes to ensure greater conditioning, flexibility, stamina, etc. Cardo is good for all ages, but of course with the proper supervision to ensure greater results. Cardo is excellent for healthy arteries, lungs, heart, and to improve you overall well being.

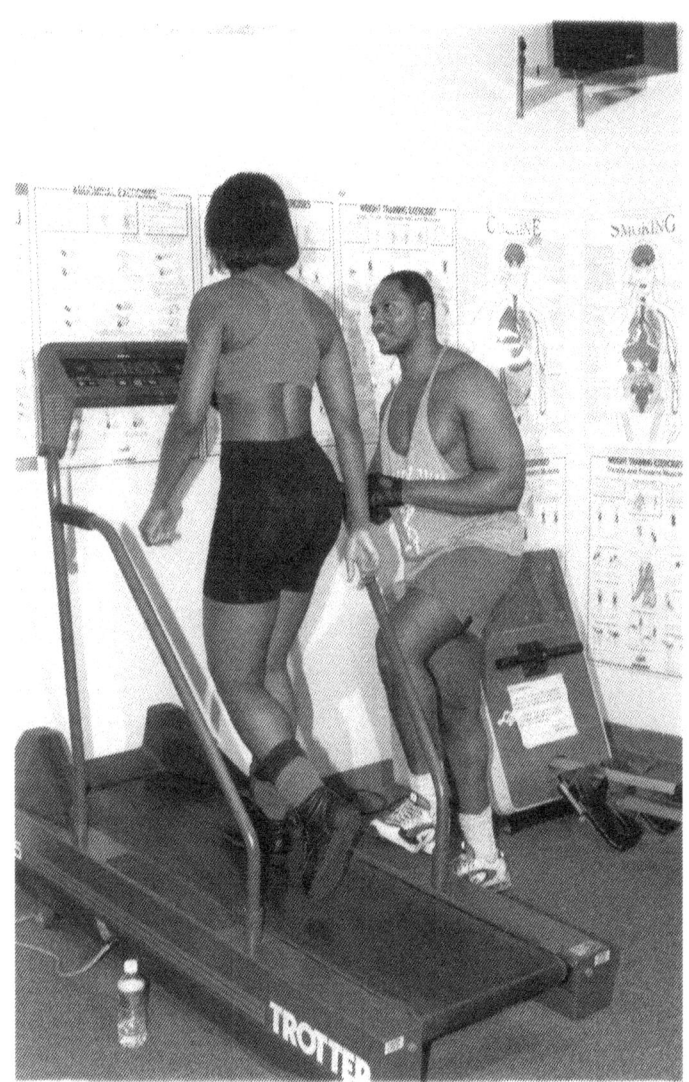

THREE-WAY INTESTINAL CLEANSING

There are so many unsafe unnatural items on the market that people are thinking twice about using certain products, but you have to use something other than water to cleanse your system thoroughly. So if you want to try some healthier ways here are some choices:

1st choice: Herbal laxative blend tea.

Note: This can be taken in the morning or at night.

2nd choice: Aloe vera gel or juice.

Note: This may be taken with 16 oz. of spring water or any of your favorite fruit juices. This is also great for people with a stomach ulcer.

3rd choice: This can be done any day of the week or weekend; for example:

Monday morning: 1 quart of water/fruit

Monday afternoon:1 quart of water/fruit

Monday evening: 1 quart of water/salad and
fruits

Eat nothing else after that.

Note: You may use vinegar and oil or lemon and oil as a salad dressing topping.

This is also an excellent way to start an exercise program, by cleansing your system free of toxic waste.

Paul J. Godfrey

PART II

Paul J. Godfrey

CHAPTER SIX

THE FREEHANDED WAY

To start off anything, you want the basics, and when it comes to setting a good foundation, free handed exercises are the perfect way to begin body building. You can do these exercises without expensive gym equipment right at home.

You will need only a few pieces of furniture and your own body weight. I realized how effective these exercises were when I alternated them with my weight training routine. They were exercises like close-grip, chin-ups, push-ups with elevation; leg raises, sit-ups, squats. It takes about three (3) to six (6) months to see how your body will be well toned and in better condition. Free hand exercises have a tonic effect on the muscles and internal organs. They gently tone and stimulate the circulatory system.

Freehand exercises shape and muscularize the body in a unique way; all of the world's best built men have included them in their workouts. Free hand exercise helps build muscle size, gives definition and creates a sculptured look.

I've outlined a program for those who are just beginning and for others who are a little more advanced. For example: Let's say you body weight is 120 pounds: You will be using the 120 pounds for resistance training. Certain exercises you can do, such as push-ups, give you the same results you'd get from doing a bench press with 120 pounds of steel plates. These are exercises that can be done basically anywhere.

Starting your exercise program

Most people, because of work or school, find it more convenient to exercise in the late afternoon or evening or in the early morning before going to work. It doesn't matter when you train, good progress can still be made.

I've discovered that training in the morning was not one of my strong points, even though my body recuperated well and my mind was focused. So I work out in the late afternoon, from two to four.

Building pre-workout energy:

The idea is to have enough carbohydrates about an hour or two before training, such as: Fruit, protein drink or an energy bar which is low in fat and fiber; this way the body is not too sluggish which can cause slow digestion. you should also have a good amount of water before, during and after training.

Designing a diet for athletes:

1. In designing a diet, it is necessary to know the person's blood pressure, body weight, body fat, temperature, number of calories expended during exercise and the individual's lifestyle and taste.

2. This information is fed into a computer which analyzes the values and tells you what the athlete needs to eat and what to avoid as well as the menu proportions.

3. The computer is programmed to know the exact levels of cholesterol, uric acid, blood sugar cholesterol (HDL) and triglycerides needed to achieve great performance.

4. All of these factors will vary according to whether a person is training or actively performing daily sports. Exercising daily is also included in this regimen, 30 minutes to one hour daily, 5 times a week.

There are two rules you should remember:

1. The best time to exercise is about one hour before you eat or two hours after you have eaten a full meal.

2. Try to eat something about two hours before exercising so your energy level will be high. Never train immediately before a meal or right after one. Immediately after you eat, you stomach needs a lot of blood to digest the food; so working blood supply goes to the stomach. the result of exercising too soon will be poor digestion of your food.

Clothing:what you wear is important; you should be comfortable. It also depends on the weather and where you're doing your training. If it's warm, you should wear tank tops and shorts. If it's cool you clothing should still be comfortable and loose. If you wear two sweatshirts they should be loose enough to move around in. Try to get cotton fabrics, they absorb sweat better than polyester and artificial fibers.

<u>Breathing</u>: breathing properly is very important when it comes to movements in exercise. If you breathe incorrectly, it could have a bad effect on your lungs and heart, because your oxygen intake will be minimized. The correct way to breathe when you train is to exhale each time you have some kind of resistance. For example: Let's say you're doing a pushup. When you press your body up from the floor, you should breathe out. <u>Remember the Rule</u>: As soon as there is any strain on your body you should breathe out. The time to inhale is when you let yourself down; when you body is under the least amount of pressure, you should always have plenty of oxygen when you train. Outdoors keeps you energy level up and lets you train longer and harder without exhaustion. With indoor training, sometimes you have to help your body get the oxygen by taking Vitamin E.

After your workouts always practice jogging, swimming. stretching which is good to prevent becoming musclebound. In fact these first set of free hand exercises could be done outdoors anywhere.

<u>Pushups</u>: The first exercise is the pushup. This is excellent for the chest, shoulders and the back of the arms (triceps). There's something I want to stress in the beginning: Do not try for high repetitions in the hopes of getting faster results! Put it out of your mind. Just remember this: Form is the most important thing when it comes to doing an exercise correctly; that counts for everything. That's why I introduced the basic exercises first. If you start doing the basic free hand exercises without any problems and without cheating, then you'll go on into weight training without cheating. Even if you can do only one pushup that's fine, as

long as it's done correctly. I am positive a week later, you'll be able to do three, six and eventually ten.

Place both hands approximately 18 inches apart (or) shoulder width. Hold your body perfectly straight and exhale as you push your body up until your arms are straight - pause - inhale, as you lower body to the floor allowing only your chest to touch. Your stomach should still be an inch or two off the floor when you touch with your chest, because your toes lift the body up a bit.

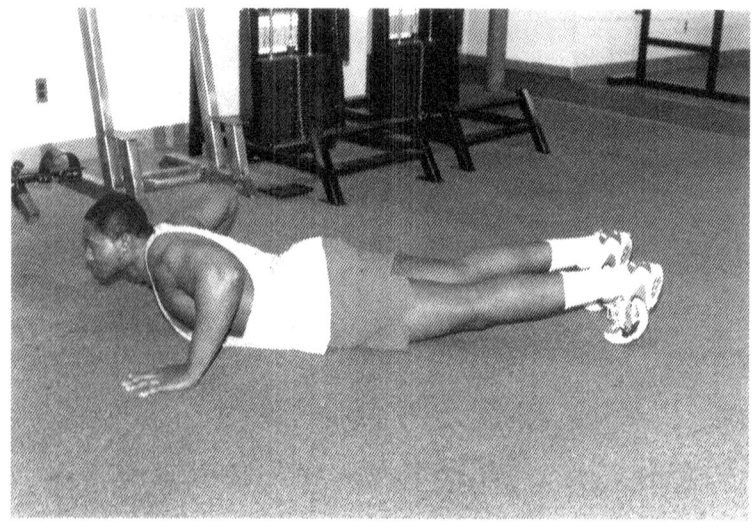

The most important thing is not to touch the floor with your stomach, or your knees and press up until your arms are locked straight. The motion should be smooth and steady while going up and down. Later you can use different hand positions to stimulate different muscle areas. For instance, if you start turning your hands toward the inside it will work more in the triceps and deltoid area, less to the pecs. Don't worry about the sets or repetitions in the beginning; within a few weeks you should work up to a total of 50 repetitions. Try 10 five times, or 5 ten times. Remember to observe strict form. If you have no problem doing so than try 100. If you can do a lot of reps easily and want more resistance, elevate your feet using a chair at first, then a table.

<u>Bent-Leg Sit-ups</u>: This is excellent for abdominal conditioning, working mostly to tighten the upper abdomen. This is also very easy on people who have lower back problems. Put both feet under a piece of furniture, a bed or a couch (or keep your heels to the floor), and bend your legs at a 45 degree angle. Hold your hands in front of your waist with your fingers close together and go up and down. It is not necessary to lie back fully - only about three-quarters of the way - but the movement should be smooth and rhythmical. With abdominals all you need is contraction. It's actually one of the few sets of muscles we don't give a full movement. We want to flex the muscles, to compress them. Do 100 repetitions, two sets of 50. If you feel comfortable doing 100 try 150.

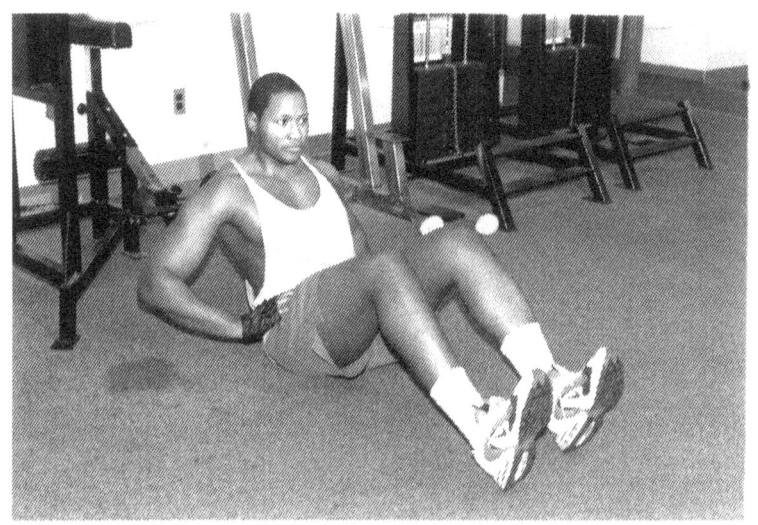

<u>Bent-Leg raises</u>: Bent leg raises warm-up the muscles of the trunk and lower back and burn the fat off the lower abdominal area. Sit-ups train the upper abdominals. I suggest leg raises with bent knees, because they're easier and you can get in more repetitions, and it's better for the back. Lie on the floor with your legs straight out, you hands under your buttocks, and you chin on your chest (this position of the head and neck causes your abdominals to flex when you're in a prone position; then pull your knees all the way into you chest area.   Remember the technique about breathing - exhale as you bring your legs up, inhale as you lower them. In this exercise, the amount of resistance is not nearly as important as how many repetitions you do.   Do a minimum of 50 repetitions.

<u>Seated Side Twists</u>: Twists are for the obliques, those muscles at the sides of the waist and for the lower back. They're a great exercise for trimming off excess fat. Put your feet under a bed, couch or any other surface that's suitable, and bend your legs at a 45-degree angle. Take both hands and twist completely to your left side, touching the floor. This should be done very smoothly and rhythmically. Do at least 50 repetitions and work up to more.

<u>Deep Knee Bends (squats)</u>: Squats will build up your thighs and strengthen your hips. They can be done in different ways. One way is to stand with your heels on a book, go all the way down, and come all the way up. The other is to stand flatfooted on the floor and go all the way up and down. I suggest for anyone to use a book for starters then eventually when you get used to doing the squats a little better, you can go on to doing the thrust squats which I have done for years as a wrestler for stamina, strength and speed, not so much for size. For any exercise you do, stand with you feet 12 to 15 inches apart either with your hands on your hips or free down to your sides. Squat down until you thighs are parallel to the floor, then raise your self slowly up again. Remember to keep your body upright and you back straight throughout the exercise. Breathe

deeply - inhaling as you squat, exhaling as you come back up - keeping your chest high and square. The same matter is done for the thrust squat, but the only difference is that it's done more rapidly with both hands clapping as you go up and down. Do 50 to 100.

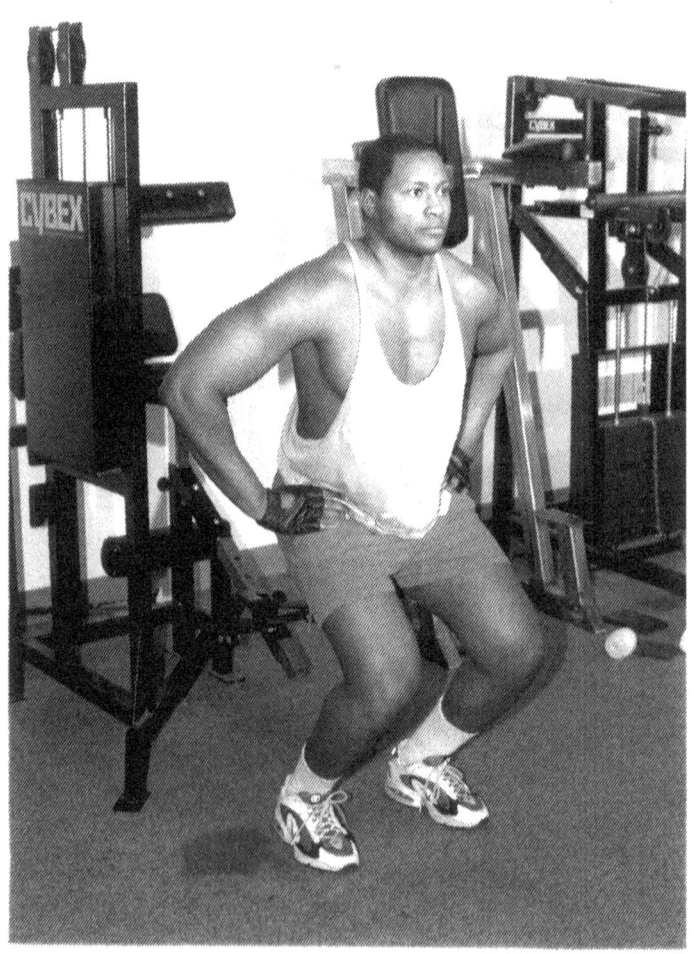

The Cobra Touch: I named this the cobra touch because it really contracts, crunches and squeezes the abdominal muscles to burn the fat off the upper and lower abdominal areas. Lie on the floor with your legs straight in the air, while holding your legs steady. Reach for both feet and lift yourself forward with both hands to touch your feet. Do a minimum of 50 repetitions.

Paul J. Godfrey

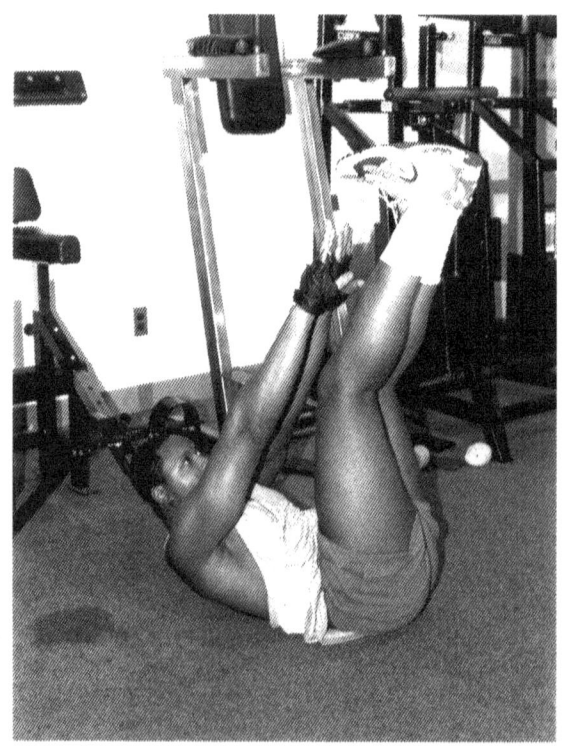

<u>The Good morning Stretch</u>: I am sure you are wondering why this exercise is called the good morning stretch. Well, for one thing, it can be done not only in the morning, but at any give time of the day or whenever you want to stretch before your workout. Take a broomstick and put it behind your neck, gripping it wide with your hands. Hold your legs stiff, your feet about shoulder width apart and bend forward until you feel a stretch in your lower back and hamstring muscles; then come up looking straight ahead. Do at least 30-50 repetitions.

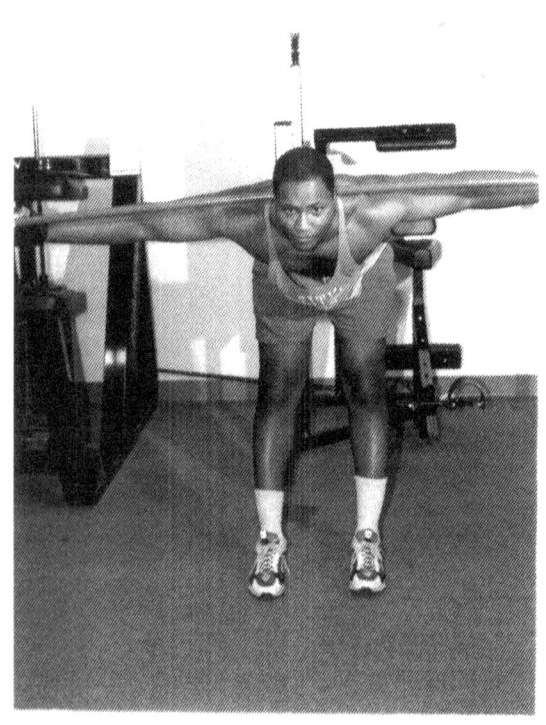

Close-Grip Chins: This is another great exercise that is good for the biceps. All you need is a chinning bar, which you can buy inexpensively that fits between doorjambs. Take an underhand grip, palms facing toward your body on the chinning bar, with the hands about 15-20 inches apart. Starting with your arms straight, pull up until your chin is over the bar and your biceps are fully contracted. Lower your body slowly until your arms are straight. Chin-ups are not easy when you do them correctly, but you will put size on your biceps. Go all the way down and all the way up, making full movements. Stretch when you reach the bottom and pull all the way up to the chin. Do not cheat by kicking your legs to help pull your body up to the top. This throws off the full benefits of the exercise. Do as many repetitions as possible, trying for a total of 25-30.

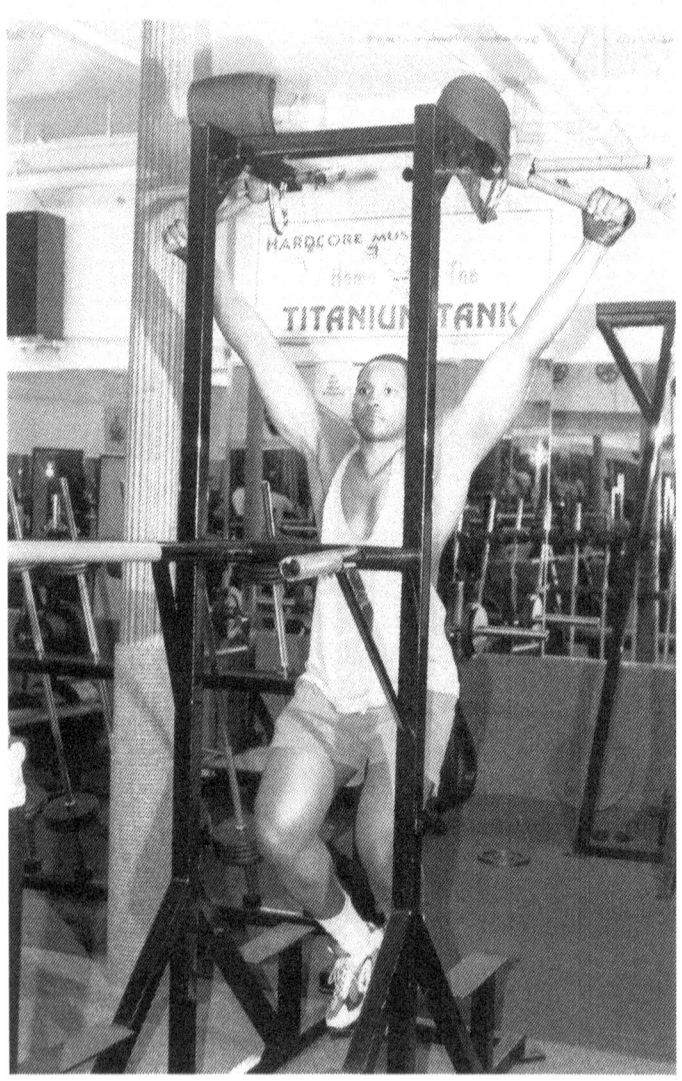

Standing Calf Raises: Unfortunately, the calves are difficult to develop, because they are made of dense muscle fibers that must really be worked to see good results. Try this exercise standing on a calve machine or the edge of your bathtub. Standing forward or reversed, raise onto your toes as high as possible and then lower your heels as slowly as possible, stretching the calf muscles on the way down; then raise all the way up again and repeat. Do 10-12 repetitions.

Paul J. Godfrey

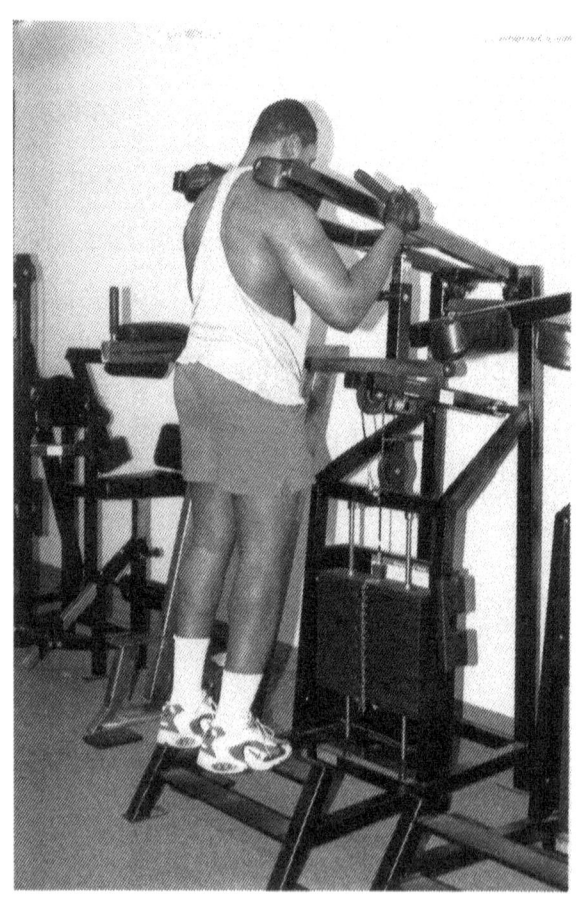

<u>Biceps/Triceps Toner</u>:   Take a broom stick or any other stick you can find that's a little taller than your own height.   Place both hands on the ends of the stick or almost near the ends and place it behind your neck and begin pulling left and right with a firm grip; if you stand in front of a mirror you can actually see how your biceps and triceps are being worked.   Try doing 50 repetitions.

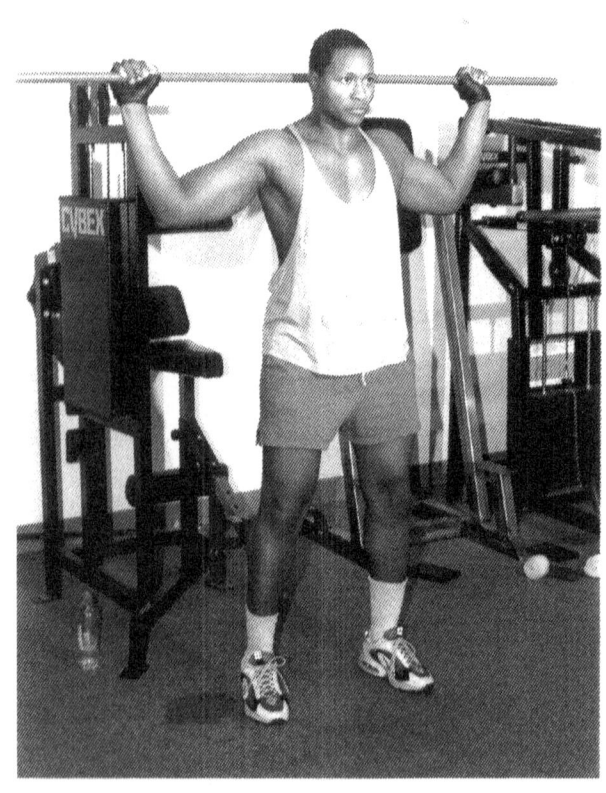

<u>The hips and buttocks toner</u>:   This is a great exercise to tone the hips and buttocks and also the lower lumbar region (spinal) part of the back. Lie flat on your back with your hands to your sides, your knees should be bent with your feet flat on the floor; bracing yourself, begin lifting your hips off the floor, pushing to contract the buttocks muscles and the lower back muscles.   It's important to do this exercise with a full smooth motion. Do 25 repetitions working up to 50.

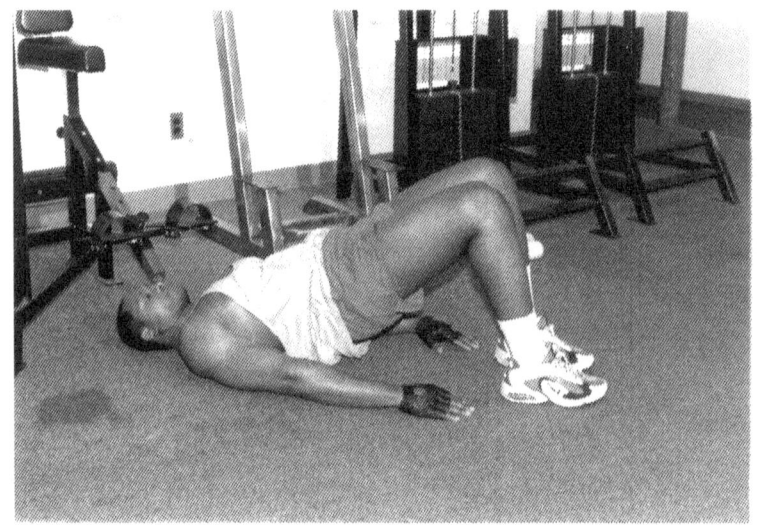

CHAPTER SEVEN

THE THREE DAY WAY TO FITNESS & NUTRITION

Body Part

(Day 1)

Quads: hack squats, leg presses, leg extensions

Hamstrings: lying leg curls, stiff leg deadlifts

Calves: standing and seated calf raises

(Day 2)

Back: pulldowns, dumbbell rows, seated rows

Shoulders: upright rows, side laterals

Abdominals: crunches, hanging leg raises

(Day 3)

<u>Chest:</u> dumbbell flyes dumbbell presses, incline barbell presses

<u>Biceps:</u> preacher curls, alternate dumbbell curls

<u>Triceps:</u> press downs, kickbacks

* NOTE: These exercises are for intermediate or advanced levels only.

<u>Bent-arm dumbbell flys</u>: Flys stretch the rib cage and build the outer pectorals. Lie flat on your back on the bench, lift your legs up and lock them in a cross position; this will eliminate strain on your stomach. Starting with a pair of dumbbells held at arms length over the chest, bend your arms slightly to take the pressure off your elbows and lower the weights out to the sides as far as you can (almost near the floor) while inhaling as much air

as possible. Then slowly raise your arms — exhaling and tensing the pectorals as you do — until the dumbbells are about 10 inches apart. At the top, flex your pectoral muscles and press the weight really hard. The idea is to make a wide circle with the dumbbells. Do three (3) sets of 8-10 repetitions.

Wide Grip Chins: Wide grip chins widen the lats and work on the entire shoulder girdle. It primarily develops the upper and outer regions of the lats and expands the scapula making it easier to widen the lats. Using a wide grip, pull yourself up until your chin is over the bar then lower the body slowly and give the lats a good stretch on the way down. Try three (3) sets of 10 repetitions or 30 straight.

Calf raises/machine/standard: Standing calf raises work on the inside, outside, lower and upper parts of the calves to give them thickness and width. The normal position is to stand on the wooden block at the base of the machine, with your toes pointed straight forward. Situate your shoulders under the padded bars and lift as high as you can on your toes. Let yourself down slowly allowing your heels to drop as far below the platform as possible. You should feel the stretch in your calves until it burns. Th mistake people make is using too much weight then they cannot observe the strict form. When the weight gets heavy it is difficult to get all of the repetitions out. Some people bend their knees using their thigh muscles to complete the exercise. This is incorrect. The right way to do the exercise for better results is to keep the knees locked, then let your heels down as far as possible and go up until the calf is fully flexed. Since the calves are a very dense muscle they need more work so go for five (5) sets of 12 repetitions.

<u>Sit-ups</u>: With knees bent — the stomach is a very noticeable body part whether it is in shape or out of shape. It is very delicate; it aids in digestion and elimination. But the key to keeping it well toned and trim would consist of eating the proper foods and using a slant board doing three sets of 50 repetitions.

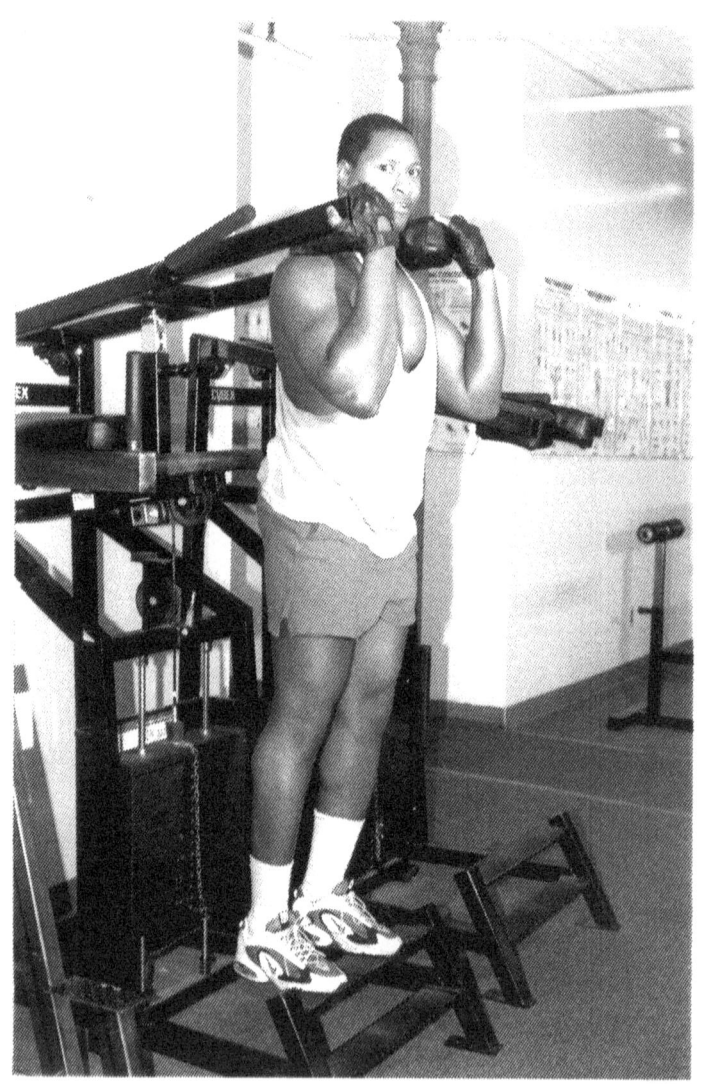

CHAPTER EIGHT

MUSCLE TENSION, BACK PAIN AND CELLULITE

I am sure everyone has experienced some sort of muscle disorder one time or another, and the only thing that was done to ease the pain was to take two aspirin or tylenol and a hot soak in your favorite formula figuring this would be sufficient to make you feel more comfortable, but sometimes you need other ideas or remedies that will thoroughly work.

For example, for people with muscle tension in the hamstrings: Put one foot in front of the other, bend forward, touching your toes with your fingertips holding this position for a count of five or longer depending on how quick your muscles respond. Repeat the same thing for the other leg. Then take a hot bath in some herbal bath salt. Soak for 15-20 minutes. Then get a rub down with Fusho Oil & Balm or Tiger Balm or use a rolling pin to relieve the pressured areas.

Back Pain: Take a hot bath in epsom or herbal bath salts for 20 minutes then use a rolling pin to thoroughly relax the entire back. Also use Fusho Oil and Balm or Tiger Balm as a finishing touch. Before bed time have a cub of Brigham Herbal Tea.

Cellulite: What is Cellulite? Cellulite is a combination of fat globules, waste matter and water imprisoned in connective tissue. Its appearance is due to strands of fibrous tissue anchored to the skin, pulling the skin inward and in the process, plumping the fat cells outward. Cellulite is something you can try to avoid, through exercise and by keeping your weight normal. But if you already have this problem, you might want to try some of the following remedies:

A. <u>Lose Some Weight</u>: Since cellulite is fat, excess weight can contribute to it. Hopefully some of what you lose will be cellulite.

B. <u>Eat Well</u>: Eat a healthy balanced diet. Eat plenty of fresh fruits and vegetables and drink fruit and vegetable juice. Drink plenty of water, at least six to eight glasses of bottled water per day. For water retention, try drinking watermelon juice of lemon juice with lecithin. All of these things will help minimize cellulite and also help detoxify your body.

C. <u>Relaxing Soak</u>: Relax in your tub with a solution containing sea salt. For smooth-feeling skin, add two cups of sea salt to warm water and soak for twenty minutes.

D. <u>Avoid</u>: Salt, which contributes to water retention and adds to cellulite problems. Stay away from coffee, cigarettes and alcohol. These substances constrict your blood vessels and may actually make your cellulite more prominent.

E. <u>Skin Techniques</u>: Dry brush your skin. It helps to improve circulation. Press a soft bristle brush gently onto your skin and rotate it in circular movements from head to toe or on cellulite areas alone. Massage trouble spots with a kneading massage in areas such as your thighs and the insides of your knees.

F. <u>Muscle Tone</u>: Building stronger muscles with methods such as nautilus or working out with weights may help fill out the tissue in cellulite problem areas.

G. <u>Stay Calm</u>: Cellulite builds up when muscles get tense; and muscles get tense when they are feeling stressed, so try to relax.

CHAPTER NINE
EATING TO STAY FIT

To stay in good shape, internally and externally, one of the best ways to achieve that is to eat good foods that are well balanced in protein, carbohydrates and fats. An exercise program is not enough. Exercise merely tones and develops existing muscles. In order to build muscles we must have the nutrients that promote growth. <u>Protein</u> is for growth, maintenance and repair of muscle tissue. Protein is the major component of your hair, nails and blood. Protein also helps regulate the water balance and metabolism of your body. Protein consists of 22 elements known as amino-acids; the human body can produce 14 of these elements, but the other eight must be obtained from poultry, eggs, fish, milk and milk products.   <u>Carbohydrates</u> are the body's main source of energy. It raises the blood sugar level and supplies the muscles with energy. You need a certain amount of carbohydrates to fuel your system so it can utilize its available protein to the greatest advantage. Without carbohydrates, your central nervous system slows down, you become sluggish and irritable. <u>Fats</u> - your body needs a certain amount of at in order to be healthy. If you deprive yourself of fat you will be unable to absorb vitamins A, E and D and the mineral calcium.

Aside from <u>protein</u>, <u>carbohydrates</u> and <u>fats</u>, you should have adequate vitamins and minerals. It is better to get our vitamins and minerals from the foods you eat. These are the vitamins your body needs to maintain itself properly:

1. <u>Vitamin A</u>: Important for good vision, skin texture and maintaining the delicate linings of the nose and throat. Sources: Carrots, milk, eggs, spinach and liver.

2. <u>Vitamin B complex</u>: Twelve B vitamins, including niacin, riboflavin and thiamine — essential to a good balance of the nervous system and the normal functioning of the digestive system. Sources: eggs, whole grains, poultry, green vegetables, fish, fruit, milk and brewers yeast.

3. <u>Vitamin C</u>: Promotes healing, builds up resistance to infection, aids in the production of connective tissues; generally strengthens the skeletal and vascular systems. Sources: Citrus fruits, tomatoes and green vegetables.

4. <u>Vitamin D</u>: Essential for strong teeth and bones. Sources: Milk, fish, eggs, chicken livers and direct sunlight.

5. <u>Vitamin E</u>: Contributes to the functioning of the circulatory, respiratory and reproductive systems. Sources: Wheat germ, vegetable oils, eggs and leafy green vegetables. In addition to vitamins, your body still requires adequate amounts of the following minerals: Calcium, magnesium, phosphorus, iron, iodine, potassium, sodium, copper, since and manganese.

I want to point out something about calcium. Calcium is a vital nutrient in the diet. You can still get an adequate amount of calcium from your food while still consuming a lowfat, low cholesterol diet you might ask why is calcium so important. Calcium is a major component of bones and teeth. When you include an adequate amount of calcium in your diet you help reduce the risk or delay the onset of osteoporosis in later life. Osteoporosis is a disease that leaves bones porous and fragile. While it affects mostly women, it can affect men as well. How much calcium is required. The United States Government recommends a minimum of 800 to 1200 milligrams of calcium daily; however, most doctors feel that to be on the safe side 1500 milligrams should be consumed daily. With a proper diet and exercise, your chances are great to pass over the possibility of thinning and weakening bones.

The use of salt and sodium with moderation

Table salt contains sodium and chloride; both are essential in the diet. However, most people eat more salt and sodium than they need. Food and beverages containing salt provide most of the sodium in our diets, much of its added during processing and manufacturing.

To moderate the use: Use salt sparingly when planning a meal. For example: Fresh and plain frozen vegetables prepared without salt are lower in sodium than ready-to-eat cereals. Milk and yogurt are lower in sodium than most cheeses. Excess sodium causes water retention, which makes you appear a few pounds fatter, but this excess water can be eliminated in about one week by dropping your sodium level.

Water: This is one element that's not favored by millions of people all over the world. But then there are some who love water despite the fact that they feel they will retain most of it if they drink too much of it. Water flushes out your system. Every time you drink a glass of water you are giving your internal organs a good cleansing. Eight 8-ounce glasses of plain water is sufficient. Water is also great for healthier looking skin and to curb your appetite. To curb your appetite, drink a glass of water before breakfast, lunch, dinner and before bedtime. This is why high — protein/low carbohydrate diets are not good. When denied carbohydrates, the body loses water (because carbohydrates hold water) and begin eating the walls of the muscle tissue. But the fat remains, and your body weight goes down because of the water and muscle loss and once you stop the diet, your overall body frame is higher in fat than before. Your weight goes up again as soon as you regain the lost water and starts building up more fat again.

There are three types of carbohydrates:

1. Processed: Avoid processed carbohydrates; they are full of sugar. They are sucrose, glucose, dextrose, maltose, fructose, lactose, sorbitol and xylitol. Bleached flour is also a processed carbohydrate. All of these sugars raise your blood level too quickly, and you get a burst of energy, but in less than a half an hour later, you blood sugar level drops. Then you crave for more sugar; and in the end, you consume many empty calories, and you gain weight.

2. Simple carbohydrates: These are found in all fruits - when you eat fruit, carbohydrates go directly to your blood stream and you get and immediate shot of energy. But as opposed to processed carbohydrates, you don't go back for more 30 minutes later.

3. Complex/Carbohydrates/Fiber: The only foods that contain dietary fiber are whole grains, fruits and vegetables. Fiber helps prevent cancer, eliminates fat from your system and provides some free calories. Free calories you might say! This is how it works: When calories are calculated for a given complex carbohydrate, the calories of the fiber content of that food are included in the calculation. The body cannot digest fiber because our intestines lack the enzymes required to break down these

rough substances. Since most complex carbohydrates consist of about 10% fiber, you actually get 10 percent worth of free calories when you consume a complex carbohydrate.

You need more than 40 different nutrients for good health. Essential nutrients include vitamins, minerals, amino acids from protein certain fatty acids from fat and sources of calories (Protein, carbohydrates and fat). These nutrients should come from a variety of foods, not from a few highly fortified foods or supplements. Any food that supplies calories and nutrients can be part of a nutritious diet.

One way to assure variety, is to choose foods each day from five major food groups, which are:

Food Group	Suggested Servings
Vegetables	3 to 5 servings
Fruits	2 to 4 servings
Breads, cereals, rice and pasta	6 or more servings
Milk, yogurt and cheese	2 to 3 servings

*Note: Some people may need more because of their body size and activity level. Young children should have a variety of foods but may need small servings.

Choose a diet low in fat, saturated fat and cholesterol. The higher levels of saturated fat and cholesterol in our diets are linked to our increased risk for heart disease. A diet low in fat makes it easier for you to include the variety of foods you need for nutrients without exceeding your calorie need because fat contains over twice the calories of an equal amount of carbohydrates or protein. A diet low in saturated fat and cholesterol can help maintain a desirable level of blood cholesterol. For adults this level is below 200 mg/dl. As blood cholesterol increases above this level, greater risk for heart disease occurs. Risk can also be increased by high blood pressure, cigarette smoking, diabetes.

What is cholesterol? Cholesterol is a substance contained in certain foods. You cannot smell, taste or see it. It is not present in plant food such as fruits and vegetables. Cholesterol is found in all foods that come from animals. Every time you eat fatty meats such as beef or pork, or anything made of whole milk, you take in cholesterol. Egg yolks are the highest source of cholesterol in the typical

American Diet. Although fish and poultry also contain cholesterol, they are lower in fat than red meat. Cholesterol is important for your general good health, and your body, in fact, can make all the cholesterol you need. However, when your diet is too high in cholesterol and saturated fat, fatty deposits can build up on the walls inside your arteries. If this continues, the arteries may become clogged. It will then be harder for your blood to get through to your heart. This matter will eventually lead to a heart attack. To help prevent such occurrences use fats and oils sparingly in cooking. Also take vitamins C, E and Lecithin to clear the arteries.

Use More	Use Less
Corn Oil	Beef Fat
Safflower Oil	Butter
Sunflower Oil	Lard
Soybean Oil	Bacon Fat
	Hydrogenated
	Margarines and
	Shortening

Helpful Garlic Solutions:

1. (Cholesterol Reducer): Garlic is excellent for blood cholesterol and can lower your cholesterol level to at least 9 percent - 1/2 to one whole.

2. (Artery Defense): Garlic capsules are also a great way to lower your cholesterol level and oxidize your blood stream to prevent heart attacks, strokes and clogging.

3. (Blood Thinner): Garlic compounds help thin the blood. Raw garlic - about three cloves a day will help improve clot-dissolving activity. Do not cook the garlic for this purpose because it will kill the strength.

4. (Infection Fighter): Garlic helps fight viruses from colds and the flu. This is also great if you have a sore throat coming on, and to prevent a cold from occurring. Garlic is also a decongestant; garlic revs up your immune system by stimulating infection fighting T-cells.

Cancer Preventive Foods:

Cancer is a very deadly disease and it can spread through your whole body at times. It can be slow moving or fast moving. But sometimes there is a chance to keep cancer at bay. Try some of these foods.

1. Cabbage: Cabbage has cancer fighting chemicals called indoles to fight off, as well as burn of a form of estrogen. When purchasing cabbage at your supermarket, avoid precut cabbage halves and quarters; the vitamin C content is lost once it is exposed.

2. Brussel Sprouts: Similar to cabbage the factors exist in reference to its chemical indoles. Buy

brussel sprouts that are small, firm and dark green - not yellow.

CHAPTER TEN

VITAMINS, MINERALS & HERBS

Here are some suggested Herbal Dietary
Supplements:

Heart: Herb combinations: cayenne, garlic
berry syrup, rejuvenaid. Single Herbs: cayenne,
hawthorn berries, common sage and yarrow.

Blood Purifier: Herb combinations: red clover
comb, vascuaid. Single Herbs: red clover, burdock
root, garlic echinacea, devil's claw chaparral.

Digestion: Herb combinations: Comfrey-
pepsin comfrey plus. Single herbs: Papaya leaves,
fennel, catnip, aloe vera juice, comfrey,
chamomile.

<u>Blood   Pressure/Circulation</u>:   Herb combinations: cayenne-garlic, vascuaid.   Single herbs: garlic alfalfa, hawthorn berry, cayenne, siberian ginseng parsley.

<u>Bowel</u>: Herb combinations: nataralax.   Single herbs: cascara sagrada, alfalfa leaves, kelp, psyllium seed, turkey rhubarb root, garlic.

<u>Colds/flu</u>:   Herb combinations: Herbalenza, herbal composition, herbal cough syrup.   Single herbs: garlic, red raspberry, parsley, white willow bark.

<u>Cough</u>:   Herb   combinations: Breathe-ease, Fenu-comf, herbal cough syrup.   Single herbs: garlic, yarrow, alfalfa, chickweed, cayenne.

<u>Hayfever/Allergies</u>:   Herb combinations: Has, rejuvenaid, fenu-thyme.   Single herbs: alfalfa, Brigham Tea, chapparal, burdock root.

Tendinitis/Bruises/Sprains: Herb combinations: Fusho oil and balm, Herbal mineral (mk-9). Single herbs: Comfrey root or leaf, kelp, dandelion, alfalfa, cayenne, arnica, horse tail grass, tiger balm.

Diuretic/Water Retention: Herb combinations: garlic-parsley, vascuaid KB Herbal Diuretic. Single herbs: parsley, juniper berries, marshmallow root, dandelion root, kelp, garlic, alfalfa leaves.

Glands: Herb combinations: IGL, IF, GL. Single herbs: Alfalfa, golden seal root, echinacea, mullein, black walnut, kelp, lobelia, licorice root.

Insomnia: Herb combinations: Hops-valerian plus, ex-stress (EZ), sleep tight tea. Single herbs: Lady's slipper root, valerian root, hops, passion flower.

Memory: Herb combinations: Remem, Rejuvenaid, Single herbs: Gotu Kola, Siberian or Korean ginseng, periwinkle, Fo-ti, Blessed Thistle, cayenne.

Weight Loss: Herb combinations: Herbal Slim, T Comb; Adrenaid. Single herbs: Chick weed, kelp, burdock root, parsley, dandelion peppermint.

Ulcer: Herb combinations: Myrrh-goldenseal plus, comfrey plus. Single herbs: comfrey leaves, myrrh gum, aloe vera juice, cayenne, alfalfa.

Nervous tension: Herb combinations: Ex-stress (EZ), sleep-tight tea, hops valerian plus. Single herbs: Licorice Root, valerian root, catnip, scullcap, cayenne.

Muscle cramps: Herb combinations: Elderberry ext, herbal mineral (mk-9) fusho oil and balm. Single herbs: Horse tail grass, oat straw, alfalfa, kelp, saffron, dong quai, tiger balm.

Menstrual: Herb combinations: Fem-mend (FC), change-o-life (MP). Single herbs: Black cohosh, blessed thistle, red raspberry squaw vine, dong quai.

Menopause: Herb combinations: Change-op/-life (MP), rejuvenaid, fem-mend (FC). Single herbs: Dong quai, licorice root, cedar berries, black cohash, damiana, kelp, siberian ginseng, alfalfa.

Sexual: Herb combinations: APH, rejuvenaid. Single herbs: Damiana, licorice root, fenugreek seed, sarsaparilla, all ginsengs.

Pancreas/Blood Sugar: Herb combinations: PC, HIGL, rejuvenaid. Single herbs: Cedar berries, garlic, Siberian Ginseng, cayenne, licorice root, golden seal root, dong quai.

Skin blemishes: Herb combinations: Red clover combination, change-o-life, AKN, BF&C, LG. Single herbs: Burdock root, dandelion root, Echinacea, kelp, alfalfa.

Vision: Herb combinations: Herbal eyebright combination. Single herbs: Eyebright, golden seal, chamomile, witch hazel.

Tiredness/Lack of Energy: Herb combinations: Ginseng gotu kila plus, rejuvenaid, PC, Adren-aid, wake-up-right tea, afternoon delight tea. Single herbs: Cayenne, yellow dock, siberian ginseng, licorice root, garlic.

Stiffness/Aching Joints: Herb combinations: Rheum-aid (Yucca-AR), fusho oil and balm, BF&C ointment, rejuvenaid. Single herbs: Devil's claw chapparal, alfalfa, brigham tea, black cohosh, comfrey, tiger balm.

Helpful Garlic Solutions

(Cholesterol Reducer) garlic is excellent for blood cholesterol and can lower your cholesterol level to at least 9 percent - 1/2 to one whole.

(Artery defense) garlic capsules are also a great way to lower your cholesterol level and oxidize your blood stream and prevent heart attacks, strokes and clogging.

(Blood thinner) garlic compounds help thin the blood. Raw garlic - about three cloves a day will help improve clot-dissolving activity. Do not cook the garlic for this purpose because it will kill the strength.

(Infection Fighter) garlic helps fight viruses from colds and the flu. This is also great if you have a sore throat coming on; and you can prevent a cold from occurring. Garlic is also a decongestant; garlic revs up your immune system by stimulating infection fighting T-cells.

CHAPTER ELEVEN

TO BECOME AND STAY STRONG
MENTALLY

1. Think before you make any decisions no matter what they are.

2. Evaluate your weaknesses from head to toe, to prevent negative happenings.

3. Don't be a softy when you should be a toughy.

4. Don't show others you are weak like they are. This will cause you to be leaned upon and possibly used.

5. If there are things you need to talk about, let it out but be careful what you say and how you say it, to keep control of yourself.

6. Never fear another human creature, only God because you don't know what to expect from him.

7. Don't do what you don't feel like doing for anyone.

8. Always keep a positive attitude.

9. Think and look further ahead, this is very important.

10. Don't do for others what others won't do for you.

11. Take on only what you can handle mentally and physically.

12. Never let you body lead you, only your mind.

13. When under stress, exercise, jog, meditate, or take a relaxing soak and sleep.

Not only will this help you mentally but this will also help you when it comes to your training program!

Peace & Love Always;

Paul J. Godfrey

About the Author

Paul Joseph Godfrey is a former model of 12years, a father of one child, an actor from H.B. Studios, and a marathon runner who finished 6 races at 4:50 time.

He is a bodyguard and special undercover agent for several celebrities, a wrestler/martial artist, fitness trainer, and sports nutritionist; also a nursing assistant, and dental assistant graduate.

He is an all around sportsman in football, wrestling, basketball etc.

Mr. Godfrey received best physical male athlete awards in high school and college. He also performed standup comedy at the Improv, overall a great guy who anyone would like!